Bogdan Alexandru Hagiu

Physical therapy in respiratory diseases

Bogdan Alexandru Hagiu

Physical therapy in respiratory diseases

LAP LAMBERT Academic Publishing

Impressum / Imprint

Bibliografische Information der Deutschen Nationalbibliothek: Die Deutsche Nationalbibliothek verzeichnet diese Publikation in der Deutschen Nationalbibliografie; detaillierte bibliografische Daten sind im Internet über http://dnb.d-nb.de abrufbar.

Alle in diesem Buch genannten Marken und Produktnamen unterliegen warenzeichen-, marken- oder patentrechtlichem Schutz bzw. sind Warenzeichen oder eingetragene Warenzeichen der jeweiligen Inhaber. Die Wiedergabe von Marken, Produktnamen, Gebrauchsnamen, Handelsnamen, Warenbezeichnungen u.s.w. in diesem Werk berechtigt auch ohne besondere Kennzeichnung nicht zu der Annahme, dass solche Namen im Sinne der Warenzeichen- und Markenschutzgesetzgebung als frei zu betrachten wären und daher von jedermann benutzt werden dürften.

Bibliographic information published by the Deutsche Nationalbibliothek: The Deutsche Nationalbibliothek lists this publication in the Deutsche Nationalbibliografie; detailed bibliographic data are available in the Internet at http://dnb.d-nb.de.

Any brand names and product names mentioned in this book are subject to trademark, brand or patent protection and are trademarks or registered trademarks of their respective holders. The use of brand names, product names, common names, trade names, product descriptions etc. even without a particular marking in this work is in no way to be construed to mean that such names may be regarded as unrestricted in respect of trademark and brand protection legislation and could thus be used by anyone.

Coverbild / Cover image: www.ingimage.com

Verlag / Publisher:
LAP LAMBERT Academic Publishing
ist ein Imprint der / is a trademark of
OmniScriptum GmbH & Co. KG
Heinrich-Böcking-Str. 6-8, 66121 Saarbrücken, Deutschland / Germany
Email: info@lap-publishing.com

Herstellung: siehe letzte Seite /
Printed at: see last page
ISBN: 978-3-659-81526-3

Copyright © 2015 OmniScriptum GmbH & Co. KG
Alle Rechte vorbehalten. / All rights reserved. Saarbrücken 2015

Table of contents

Introduction...	5
Cap. 1. Obstructive syndrome - pathological entities and recovery...	7
Cap. 2. Restrictive lung disease...	16
Cap. 3. Physical therapy of restrictive lung disease.................	19
Cap. 4. Mixed ventilatory dysfunction......................................	23
Cap. 5. Recovery of patients with pneumoconiosis...................	26
Cap. 6. Evaluation of respiratory function...............................	27
Cap. 7. Effort testing for the respiratory apparatus................	31
Cap. 8. Physical therapy for patients with respiratory diseases..	40
Cap. 9. Respiratory gymnastics...	51
Cap. 10. Tolerance of the respiratory patient to effort............	58
References...	65

Introduction

This book constitutes the English version, with changes and additions, of the academic course headed "Kinetoterapia afecțiunilor respiratorii", Publishing House of "Alexandru Ioan Cuza" University, Iasi, Romania, (in press), author being Bogdan-Alexandru Hagiu. It is addressed to kinetotherapists. The work contains notions about respiratory diseases and their possible treatments. A special emphasis is placed on ventilatory dysfunction treatment by physical therapy.

Cap. 1. Obstructive syndrome - pathological entities and recovery

Pulmonary rehabilitation is the most widely accepted non-pharmacological method of treatment in chronic lung disease (chronic obstructive pulmonary disease, asthma, bronchiectasis) resulting in reduced breathlessness, reduce the number of days of hospitalization, increased quality of life [1].

Characteristic for the patient with OVD is the presence of airflow limitation that is based on the increase in airway resistance to the passage of air column; obstructive phenomenon can be located anywhere along the airway.

Depending on the location of airflow obstruction are differentiated upper airway obstructive syndrome (including trachea) and the obstructive syndrome of lower respiratory airflow (from main bronchi to alveoli).

In turn, mechanisms of bronchial obstruction are potentially reversible and potentially irreversible.

The mechanisms of reversible bronchial obstruction

The causes that determine reversible bronchial obstruction are varied, from functional to anatomical.

Thus, distinction is made:

Mucociliary system disorders	Mucus hypersecretion increases resistance to flow (at thicknesses greater than 300 mm). Increased mucous viscosity contributes to the installation of airflow limitation. This resistance depends directly proportional to the airflow rate. A viscous mucus secretion in the medium and large airways produce a decrease in expiratory volume in one second (even without hypersecretion) and total obstruct the small airways. Is impaired the mobility of the vibratile cilia, leading to mucociliary transport disorder, the underlying processes of other pathological phenomena.
Bronchospasm	The process can be produced by immune or neurogenic pathophysiological mechanisms mediated by vagus nerve, or due to the action of irritants directly on the bronchial mucosa. Bronchospasm is the main etiological factor of obstructive respiratory syndrome.
Bronchial mucosal	It may be the result of local allergies or infections

edema	and has the effect of reducing bronchial caliber, resulting in significant increases in flow resistance.

The pathophysiological mechanisms of bronchial obstruction (wich are reversible) may contribute to installation or even cause bronchial hyperreactivity.

Bronchial hyperreactivity is defined as an exaggerated bronchoconstrictor response of the airways to a variety of physical, chemical and pharmacological stimuli. In a normal subject not cause bronchoconstriction phenomenon.

The pathological process occurs in asthma, chronic bronchitis, emphysema.

The term of bronchial hyperactivity includes the hypersensitivity, meaning the occurrence of bronchospasm in vague excitement.

The substrate is an increased sensitivity of vagal receptors or just occurrence of an exaggerated muscular response in the presence of normal vagal reactions (in conditions of bronchial muscles hypertrophy). Bronchospasm may be produced as by the local biochemical mechanisms - release of histamine and prostaglandins, or mast cell accumulation.

The mechanisms of irreversible bronchial obstruction consist of hypertrophy and hyperplasia of secretory cells.

In the obstructive syndrome occur gland hypertrophy in the bronchial walls and hyperplasia of caliciform cells. Consequences are bronchial wall thickening and bronchiolar obstructive phenomena due to changes of epithelium, expressed by qualitative and quantitative changes of mucus secreted, adhering to its surface.

The pathophysiological mechanisms described above lay the foundation of the following conditions:

Bronchial and peribronchial fibrosis	As a result of repeated and prolonged inflammatory conditions (bacterial or viral infections, irritation of cigarette smoke) in bronchioles are formed fibrous processes causing obstruction, airway narrowing or damage.
Atrophy of the bronchial wall	The pathological process of bronchial wall interest all or some of its components (atrophy of the basal membrane, cartilage, smooth muscle, glandular structures). Those pathological processes participate especially in the establishment of airflow limitation in emphysema.
The destruction of	In emphysema and suppurative processes of

| airways | various etiologies occur damages of the bronchioles and alveoli. |

Ventilatory dysfunctions may be of restrictive or obstructive type.

Etiopathogeny of restrictive ventilatory dysfunction (RVD)	Decrease vital capacity (VC) by: - tuberculous lesions - severe emphysema - pleural symphysis - pulmonary fibrosis - pulmonary circulatory stasis - respiratory muscle paralysis - surgical procedures that results in a reduction of the lung parenchyma
Etiopathogeny of obstructive ventilatory dysfunction (OVD)	Decrease airway caliber by: - asthma - spastic bronchitis - obstructive emphysema - chronic bronchiolitis

Obstructive syndrome characterized especially chronic bronchitis, emphysema, asthma.

Chronic bronchitis and emphysema (emerged as a consequence of, or induced by the same etiological factors) make up chronic obstructive bronchitis (COPD).

Diagnosis of COPD	is based on clinical signs: chronic or recurrent productive cough lasting more than two years, at least three months per year, and/or persistent dyspnea
The diagnosis of asthma	chronic respiratory disease with paroxysmal crises of dyspnea that subside spontaneously or through treatment with bronchodilators

Chronic obstructive bronchitis (COPD) is a syndrome consisting of chronic bronchitis (pathological condition characterized by a chronic and excessive mucous secretion in the bronchial tree, is expressed clinically by coughing for at least two years for at least three months/year, and is not determined by a specific pulmonary disease) and emphysema (dilation of respiratory bronchioles with destruction of alveolar septa or walls).

Definition of emphysema are based on pathological while chronic bronchitis is diagnosed on clinical criteria. Chronic bronchitis may be complicated by a pulmonary emphysema, or may overlap this condition.

Because of the difficulties of differentiating between COPD and PE, has been introduced the following classification:
- type A clinical form of COPD - predominantly emphysematous;
- type B clinical form of COPD - predominantly bronchitis.

COPD type A	Clinical criteria: - aged 55-75 years - occasional cough - constant dyspnea - lung infections rarely occurs - radiological criteria - increased pulmonary transparency - lung drawing disappeared - flattened diaphragm - hypertransparency of retrosternally space Functional criteria: - lowering the oxygen concentration is low or moderate - sometimes there is increased concentration of carbon dioxide - BP is normal or slightly increased - chronic pulmonary heart disease installs rare - exercise tolerance is relatively good
COPD type B	Clinical criteria: - age 45-65 years - cough before installing dyspnoea - purulent sputum - variable dyspnea - frequent respiratory infections Radiological criteria: - normal or increased pulmonary transparency - normal or strengthened lung drawing - normal diaphragm Functional criteria: - lowering the concentration of oxygen (important) - increasing the concentration of carbon dioxide - often, chronic pulmonary heart disease - low exercise tolerance

Asthma is an airflows obstructive syndrome. The pathophysiologic mechanism is based on bronchospasm triggered by atopy, always being present the phenomenon of bronchial hyperactivity. Non-allergic asthma is also described.

Asthma attack can be triggered not only by the reaction antigen - antibody underlying allergic reactions, but also by bronchial infections, mental stress, effort, pollution, administration of bronchoconstrictives.

Allergic-type reactions (type I and III), outside sensitization, may be due to a parasympathetic hyperstimulation. Type I allergic reaction is triggered by the contact between an allergen from the external environment (dust, fluff, fungi, chemicals) and immunoglobulin E, respectively pathophysiological chain being conditioned by a certain genetic predisposition.

Following degranulation of mast cell histamine and serotonin are released (the chemical messengers that bronchoconstriction, edema and bronchial mucous gland secretion stimulation. Clinically, asthma is manifested by attacks of paroxysmal dyspnea, that often occur without a highlighted cause (moisture, fog, emotions, exercise, contact with different allergens or dust), often being nocturnal.

Dyspnea is the main element of the diagnosis of asthma, respiratory rate being low and exhalation prolonged. Other clinical signs are wheezing (characteristic of acute asthma), and cough, which may be dry or wet. Sputum is mucous, sticky and pearly, mucopurulent (if overlaps and infection).

Below is comprised a classification of main etiologic and clinical forms of asthma.

Extrinsic bronchial asthma (allergic, atopic)	The etiologic agent is represented by various exogenous allergens that commonly enters the body by inhalation. The pathophysiologic mechanism is immunoallergic, respectively type I hypersensitivity reaction. The condition starts between 35-45 years on the background of a preexisting atopy (the patient presents other allergic events). Clinically, extrinsic bronchial asthma is characterized by: - paroxysmal bouts of breathlessness - cough accompanied by wheezing, ceding spontaneously or after bronchodilator medication, and followed by asymptomatic intervals. - allergy tests are positive
Intrinsic bronchial	Etiopathogeny is apparently of inflammatory cause, a major role being of repeated infections. Onset of the

asthma	disease is at extreme age (under five years or after 45). Evolution and prognosis tends to be more severe comparing to other forms of asthma, also because between asthma crises remission of symptoms is incomplete.
Exercise-induced asthma	Etiopathogeny is less elucidated; this form of asthma is often associated with bronchial hyperreactivity. Exercise-induced asthma is more common in children and youth. The exercise produced a moderate bronchodilation, followed by gradual bronchoconstriction, reaching a maximum of a few minutes after exercise. The crisis appears depending on the intensity and duration of exercise, but also on its type.

Recovery of airflow limitation

Recovery is based on the stage of obstructive syndrome, ie chronic or acute stage of airflow obstruction. The first step is diagnosis (anamnesis, clinical and radiological, respiratory function tests, laboratory samples). Then the correlation with socio-professional survey will form the therapeutic and rehabilitation program.

Recovery objectives of the patient with obstructive ventilatory dysfunction are:
- removing the root causes that causes (or aggravating) the progression of obstructive ventilatory dysfunction (smoking, air pollution, alcohol)
- prevention of respiratory infections
- treatment and prevention of psychiatric disorders that may become factors of maintenance or aggravation of respiratory functional deficit
- treating nasal septum deviation
- scoliosis correction
- treatment of cardio-vascular diseases
- treatment of bronchial obstruction
- respiratory muscle toning
- progressive rehabilitation with exercises and occupational therapy
- socio-professional reintegration

The treatment of obstructive ventilatory dysfunction includes:

Characteristics of drug treatment	- there is not a strictly medical treatment, but associated with physical therapy methods - use of antibiotics and antifungal chemotherapy - infection in chronic bronchial obstruction may be permanent, but most often is episodic (occurring during acute inflammatory processes)

	- antimicrobials (tetracycline, ampicillin, erythromycin) are administered in acute episodes of obstructive ventilatory syndrome - patients take antibiotics and antifungal - mucolytics - the removal of secretions - add to this, the hygienic-dietary measures (humidification, fluid administration) - iodine is administered in the form of potassium iodide - Bromhexin hydrolyze proteins and increased lysosomal enzyme activity - corticosteroid therapy is done only in severe forms of ventilatory obstructive syndrome, when bronchospasm is present - Bronchodilators (by inhalation or orally) is given only to the deepening respiratory and only if the outcome is favorable (clinical and functional); the dose never increases - an optimal combination is Miofilin in combination with sympathomimetic sprays
Hygienic-dietary, therapeutic and educational measures	Dietary regimen consists of a balanced diet rich in vitamins, with small and often meals. Calorie food rations will be easier if the subject is overweight, low-salt due to administration of cortisone. Are to be avoided allergens (pollens and others, especially for asthmatics), respiratory infections, smoking. Physical therapy will aim at preserving the exercise capacity.
Physiotherapy	Physiotherapy of OVD underlying the recovery and consists of: - aerosol therapy - assisted ventilation - physiotherapy - oxygen - Spa treatment Physical therapy program shall be drawn based on clinical and functional status of the patient. The therapy programs are distinguished for severe forms of OVD and programs for mild forms of OVD.
Therapy in severe forms of OVD	OVD are evolving with severe forms of respiratory failure. Physical therapy has the same importance as drug therapy in the recovery

	of these patients. Firstly are necessary rest and correct positioning of the patient in bed, in order to achieve muscle relaxation and possibly achieve cough rehabilitation and bronchial drainage. Must be avoided prolonged bed rest; in case it happens, however, the patient will perform simple and limited movements, especially in the extremities. 2-4 times will be perform postural drainage in the lateral decubitus position on a horizontal plane (the patient has to cough to evacuate bronchial secretions). Expiratory flow augmentation technique can be used in combination with oxygen therapy and aerosols. Respiratory reeducation is based on abdominal breathing without changes to the rhythm and depth of respiration. It is necessary the rehabilitation to effort after bed rest, especially if it was extended, and psychotherapy, which must accompany any stage of the recovery program.
Therapy of medium forms of OVD	OVD medium forms are most prevalent in respiratory rehabilitation services. Daily physical therapy program must be executed at least once/day. After deinstitutionalization the patient must repeat the following physiotherapy elements: - posture - corrective gymnastics - controlled cough - respiratory rehabilitation - training exercise Kinetotherapy involves the following steps: - complete diagnosis (clinical and laboratory exams that evaluate the status of respiratory and cardiac function at rest and during exercise) - to learning by the patient of techniques of execution of rehabilitation procedures (number of executions, duration, intensity, breaks).

Postural drainage is useful in patients with chronic bronchitis. In the case of acute emphysema, it is necessary than in the presence of the infection.

The oxygen therapy is not without side effects; they work by interfering with physiotherapist activity.

Improvements in dyspnea in patients with COPD is followed by improved quality of life, demonstrated by specific tests [2].

Cap. 2. Restrictive lung disease

Restrictive lung disease (RLD) is characterized by pathological damage to the lung parenchyma, the airways being functional.

The pathophysiologic mechanism	Pathological processes
Factors which limit the expansion of the chest	- neuromuscular dysfunction consecutively to cranio-cerebral trauma, cerebral vascular lesions or neurasthenia, intercostal neuralgia - musculoskeletal dysfunction consecutively to thoracic kyphoscoliosis, chest fractures, ankylosing spondylitis - diaphragmatic dyskinesias consecutively to abdominal tumors, ascites, surgical interventions to the abdomen
The factors which limit the expansion of the lung	- pleural disease (pleurisy, pneumothorax) - cardio pericardial disease (pericarditis, cardiac hypertrophy); - partial destruction of elastic lung tissue (pulmonary emphysema, atelectasis, pneumonia, diffuse pulmonary stasis) - impairment of lung parenchyma: tuberculosis, pneumonia, pulmonary resections, pulmonary benign or malignant tumors

Restrictive lung disease can worsen by installing alveolar hypoventilation or overall respiratory failure, the latter being favored by poliomyelitis, kyphoscoliosis, interstitial pneumonia, tuberculosis, lung tumors.

Pathophysiological chain in the evolution of RPD include hypoxia due to alveolar hypoventilation and hypercapnia.

| Alveolar hypoventilation | It is determined by three mechanisms:
- reduction of nervous control of ventilation intensity through neurological diseases (central or peripheral)
- respiratory muscle weakness
- a marked increase of breathing labor through pulmonary or musculoskeletal (chest) diseases |

	It has the effect of modifying respiratory gas pressure in the alveoli and blood (decreased partial pressure of oxygen and increased carbon dioxide partial pressure).
Hypercapnia (increased blood carbon dioxide)	is an injury that occurs in blood chemistry and is characteristic for respiratory failure achieved by hypoventilation
Simultaneous presence of hypoxia and hypercapnia	This pathophysiological aspect triggers the compensating body's defense mechanisms, namely: - decreased blood oxygen partial pressure increases the heart rate and the number of red blood cells - increase in the excitability of the respiratory center is followed by the increase of amplitude and frequency of respiration, thereby eliminating a large amount of carbon dioxide In the early stages of respiratory failure these compensatory mechanisms maintain blood constants normal. Decompensation occurs when these mechanisms are overcome, and is characterized by the decrease in blood oxygen and increase in carbon dioxide concentration.

Kypho-scoliosis, ankylosing spondylitis, obesity, and pulmonary fibrosis produce a significant increase in ventilator labor since decreased lung elasticity requires a greater force for achieving respiratory movements. Initially, additional contraction of inspiratory muscles maintain current volume, but later a respiratory rate increase is required.

Below are the main diseases that constitutes causes of RPD.

Condition	The mechanism of induction or exacerbation of RPD
Kypho-scoliosis	Chest deformities, depending on the severity, location, presence of chest stiffness, leading to cardio respiratory failure installation. a) Kypho-scoliosis produce RPD, as evidenced by: - decrease in vital capacity - current volume dropped to 200-300 ml (compared to the normal 500 ml) - increased respiratory rate b) Ankylosing spondylitis may also cause RPD, as evidenced by:

	- decrease in vital capacity by 15-45% - lowering the maximum ventilation; - slight increase in residual volume - increased mobility of the diaphragm, whose range of movement reaches 10-15 cm (3-4 inches in quiet and 7.6 inches in forced breathing at normal individual) - hypoventilation with ventilatory failure, which occurs only if lung infections are present or obstructive respiratory syndrome is associated
Obesity	Obesity produce dyspnea even in healthy individuals, because this condition affects the respiratory control, respiratory mechanics, respiratory gas exchange and cardiovascular adaptation to effort.
Pachypleuritis	Pachypleuritis means pleural thickening, occurs in a row of local inflammation and, if extended (affects a fully hemitorace) causes a mechanical overload of thoraco-lung appliance. If pachypleuritis underlying lung is healthy, it is normal respiratory function at rest and can decompensate with exertion or in case of respiratory diseases. In the latter case RPD and OVD are associated, ie patients with COPD and pachypleuritis.
Diffuse interstitial fibrosis	It is a group of disorders that have in common interstitial lung fibrosis. This may be due to inflammation caused by bacterial, viral, parasitic, poisoning (including drugs), or may be idiopathic. Alveolar fibrosis cause alveolar edema, that results in airways sclerosis. The disorder is manifested by a decrease in the maximum quantity of oxygen. The association of chronic obstructive pulmonary disease in the late stages of the disease worsens prognosis.

Cap. 3. Physical therapy of restrictive lung disease

Except diffuse interstitial fibrosis, respiratory disorders that mechanical overload and produce alveolar hypoventilation results in final in restrictive respiratory dysfunction. Functional decompensation (decrease ventilator debit) can occur suddenly due to a respiratory infection, trauma or intense physical effort.

It is considered respiratory decompensation (and consequently acute respiratory failure) decreasing the pressure of oxygen in the arteries under 50 mm Hg and increase in blood pressure of carbon dioxide greater than 50 mm Hg.

Therapy aimed at the causes of obstructive respiratory dysfunction and increased respiratory muscle force.

| Physiotherapy of causes of mechanical overload | Treatment should be set up early, having prophylactic value. Since childhood must be made the rehabilitation of postural defects, especially scoliosis, and treatment of obesity by reduced calorie diet. Also, do gymnastics for correcting the spine position in ankylosing spondylitis. Physical therapy consists of gym, massage and electrotherapy to correct functional deficits of the thorax. It aims to increase localized expansion by techniques to promote lung ventilation in different segments and thus increase the amplitude of respiratory movements. Following is improving current volume. The exercises aim high amplitude movements principle, targeting high thoracic, axillary, medium or low regions, or even a whole hemithorax. Inspir can be increased by special positioning or by coupling upper limb or trunk movements. The expansion of some thoracic regions must be accompanied by blocking others to maximize therapeutic effect. Blocking can be achieved through manual pressure exerted by the physical therapist, by the use of straps, and in particular the posture (lateral decubitus on the side that should be blocked). The regions in which there is ventilatory |

		compensation may be identified by careful observation of respiratory movements. Depending on the condition that causing or worsening the ventilatory dysfunction, the patient can do the following exercises: - in kyphoscoliosis, spondylitis or pachypleuritis are done located expansion exercises - abdominal breathing exercises are indicated to combat obesity - interventions on fans parameters are not recommended as in patients with restrictive ventilatory dysfunction this worsens dyspnea The patient with RPD, unlike the one with OVD, tailor spontaneously their own rhythm and amplitude of breathing.	
Increasing respiratory muscle pump efficiency	Fatigue is a major factor for the installation of hypoventilation, and therefore any means which reduces labor results in improving respiratory ventilatory dysfunction. To improve respiratory muscle metabolism may be given oxygen. To increase the current volume are useful toning exercises for abdominal muscles and to improve the elasticity of the diaphragm.	
Adaptation to effort	The first sign of RPD is dyspnea on exertion, even if it occurs later than if OVD. With the onset of decompensated respiratory failure, the patient is considered disabled. The recovery methods are the same as in patients with OVD: therapeutic walk, cycle ergometer, treadmill. Training methodology differs in that it is obligatory the initial testing at dosed effort, with and without administered of oxygen.	
	Depending on the results of the test the patients will be grouped into three categories:	
	1) individuals that under oxygen administration tolerates the effort	in these patients is contraindicated any effort until drug therapy

		and physical therapy improves clinical and functional status
	2) individuals that under administration of oxygen tolerates efforts greater than 60 W	in these patients dosed effort is applied in steps, from 30-40 W, only under oxygen administration. Means are ergometer bike or treadmill. Are added an occupational therapy program with increased intensity, that do not require oxygen.
	3) patients who can perform efforts to 60 W without oxygen administration and without causing intolerance	To these patients are prescribed exercises to increase breathing muscles tone, but also of peripherals musculature
Restoring reactivity of respiratory centers and respiratory blood gas balance	The treatment of patients with RPD has the following objectives: - restoring normal blood concentrations of respiratory gases, primarily the one of carbon dioxide - correction of acidosis - increased sensitivity of the respiratory centers to chemical composition of blood It requires an hospitalization of 7-10 days,	

	during which establish: - administration of diuretics, cardiac tonics, antibiotics, bronchodilators, expectorant; shall be avoided sedatives - hygienic-dietary measures: bed rest, potassium and vitamin supplement diet, high caloric regime (excluding obese) - oxygen therapy is performed without exceeding 90% blood oxygen saturation (as otherwise there suppresses the role of hypoxemia as respiratory stimulus, which is not intended until restoring the respiratory center) - physiotherapy, consisting in gym and assisted breathing - psychotherapy The recommendation is that the patient continue rehabilitation program at home.

In the case of overlapping of conditions that decrease the force of contraction of the respiratory muscles (poisoning, coma, brain hemorrhage, polio, paralysis of the phrenic nerve, spinal injuries, myasthenia, myotonia) is installed an alveolar hypoventilation with acute respiratory failure. In this case the prognosis is grim and therapeutic approach is unique and consists of treatment of the patient in an intensive care unit that provides for mechanical ventilation.

Physical therapy will follow the prevention and treatment of muscle atrophy. Physiotherapist - neurologist collaboration is essential.

Some studies have shown the success of post-operative physical therapy for the rehabilitation of patients with small cell lung carcinoma [3].

Cap. 4. Mixed ventilatory dysfunction

Mixed ventilatory dysfunction (MVD) consists in association of restrictive and obstructive respiratory dysfunction, with the predominance of one of them. Clues to the diagnosis are: decreased vital capacity (VC) and total lung capacity (CPT), along with forced expiratory volume in 1 second (FEV_1) and Tiffeneau index. Diseases that underlie MDV development and may be recovered by physical therapy are pneumoconiosis and post-tuberculosis syndrome.

Pneumoconiosis are chronic pulmonary fibrosis processes, not systemized. They are produced by the inhalation of organic or mineral dust (silica) and pathological lesions are specific to type and quantity of powder permeated in airways. Dust accumulation in the lungs without determining fibrosis characterized pneumoconiosis of accumulation. Activation of macrophages by toxicity of inhaled particles trigger the process of fibrosis, representing sclerogenic pneumoconiosis. In clinical and etiopathogenic terms pneumoconiosis are divided into three categories.

Pneumoconiosis with small airway obstruction	anthracosis	It is an occupational disease that occurs in miners of coal mining. If pollutants contain also silica, there is a mixed pneumoconiosis - antracosilicosis. Simple anthracosis is characterized by: - increased residual volume - low or normal FEV Forms of anthracosis with massive fibrosis fall into the category of mixed ventilatory dysfunction.
	Siderosis	Siderosis is caused by the inhalation of iron ore particles. Clinical symptoms are relatively discrete.
	Byssinosis	Byssinosis is a mixed ventilatory dysfunction caused by chronic inhalation of vegetable dust (cotton, hemp). The onset is characterized by the sign called "monday fever": cough, dyspnea. Radiological examination is normal.
Pneumoconiosis	Asbestosis	Is encountered at the workers in

with increased lung elastic recoil and decreased capacity of diffusion for respiratory gases		industries that use asbestos. The inhalation of asbestos fibers causes a diffuse interstitial fibrosis that may be associated with a pleural reaction. Clinical signs of asbestosis also include nasopharyngitis, marked fatigue, headache, dizziness. Diagnosis is based on medical history and radiological examination. After exposure, asbestosis continues its evolution, even if the individual was removed from coniogen environment. Because of this treatment is that of complications (recurrent bronchopulmonary infections, chronic pulmonary heart).
	Farmer's lung	This pneumoconiosis is common at the millers and baker; the etiologic agent is the dust of moldy hay. The acute form is pneumonia and the chronic one is interstitial fibrosis. At the radiological examination is observed areas of emphysema.
Pneumoconiosis with confounding lung function disorders	Silicosis	The etiologic agent of silicosis is the particulate silicon; they are the only particles that have the ability to destroy macrophages. Clinically occur coughing and later dyspnea at effort. It is a restrictive type ventilatory dysfunction. Evolution is chronic, aggravated by overlapping og chronic obstructive pulmonary disease. The signs of advanced silicosis are highlighted on physical examination: variable chest tone, incomplete breathing, bronchial rales. With the increase of dyspnea, that comes to manifestation at small efforts, appear vague, tightness and

		intermittent chest pain, fatigue, decreased exercise capacity. Are distinguished the following clinical forms: - early silicosis (acute or "galloping"), that occurs in the case of heavy and short exposures and progresses to exitus in a few years - late silicosis, that occurs after a clinico-radiological latency of several years from occupational exposure to silica dust - unilateral silicosis, that occurs exceptionally on the background of pre-existing injuries; is due probably of certain preexisting deterioration which favors fibrosis Major complication of silicosis is tuberculosis, the association being called silicotuberculosis. Other possible complications are chronic pulmonary heart (which may occur early in the disease) and respiratory tract infections (which increase OVD).

Cap. 5. Recovery of patients with pneumoconiosis

The recovery program is determined by testing to effort, patient age, duration in years of contact with conigene dust, lung loading degree (as evidenced by X-rays). Lesions of pneumoconiosis are final and potentially evolutive (even if the patient was removed from the polluted environment).

In pneumoconiosis recovery objectives are:

Objectives	Means of achievement
Kinetoprophylaxy of occupational diseases	- exercises for back muscles - lumbar stabilization exercises - McKenzie exercises for back pain
stopping or decreasing the rate of disease progression	- establishing an early diagnosis - removing the patient from the conigen environment - identification and exclusion/treating bronchopulmonary aggressive factors (smoking, alcohol, infections) - climatic therapy (areas with high load in negative ions) - aerosol therapy - increasing immunity by training and hardening
treatment of superimposed chronic obstructive pulmonary disease	- administration of antibiotics, mucolytics, corticosteroids [4]
determining the degree of respiratory functional deficit	functional exploration of lungs - spirometry - especially highlights the decrease of vital capacity
compensation of respiratory functional shortfall	physical therapy to mobilize and eliminate the secretions

Ideal is control, disease prevention, using respiratory filters and devices for dust removal, mine ventilation, limiting working hours and the introduction of breaks.

Cap. 6. Evaluation of respiratory function

Below are systematized the steps of exploration of lung function and diseases which require them, with some elements of therapy.

to establish the diagnosis in diseases whose clinical picture is dominated by signs of pulmonary function impairment	asthma, emphysema, pulmonary fibrosis	at all stages functional explorations purpose is to establish the existence of lung function disorder, its causes and extent, and particularly the identification of respiratory failure by dosing concentrations of oxygen and carbon dioxide
assessment of pulmonary function deficiencies in an early stage	at this stage, preventive measures and/or treatment are still effective	
irreversible functional deficits assessment (establishing a functional balance)	functional balance sheet necessary for medical or surgical interventions on lungs	
time monitoring, by visual examination of the evolution of disorders identified	the step is needed to implement preventive and curative measures such as the changing working conditions or functional therapy	

Laboratory evaluation of respiratory function is made by radiological examinations and spirometry.

Circulated air volumes may be approximated by three radiographs made at the end of resting expiration, at the end of maximum inspiration and respectively at the end of maximum expiration.
Evaluation of respiratory function involves spirometry, measuring vital capacity, fan flow, flow resistance in the airways, lung elasticity, gaseous transfer through alveolar-capillary membrane.

Deep breathing, required for example to determine expiratory volume in one second (FEV_1), can trigger bronchodilation in healthy subjects, both bronchodilation and bronchoconstriction in patients with asthma, and bronchodilation in patients with obstructive ventilatory dysfunction.

For clinical cases that evolve with significant dyspnea there is the option of recording functional vital capacity with a submaximal expiratory effort.

The decrease in forced expiratory volume (FEV) occurs in case of increase airway resistance (bronchitis, asthma) or the existence of emphysema (where elasticity is much diminished). Therefore FEV determined by spirometry or pneumotachograph with integrator volume is the first choice test for the diagnosis of obstructive ventilatory dysfunction.

The mechanisms that cause decreasing airway caliber and thus decrease in FEV	Consequences of decrease FEV
- inflammation (swelling and cell infiltration) of bronchial mucosa - hypersecretion of mucus with increased viscosity - surfactant alterations in small airways - bronchospasm - airway fibrosis	- decrease of expiratory flow - reduction of elastic recoil, for example in pulmonary emphysema - reducing of respiratory muscle force - decrease in lung volume, in the restrictive conditions

Tiffeneau index or index of bronchial permeability

Tiffeneau index = FEVx100/CV

An index of bronchial permeability below 70% is pathological as denoting an obstructive syndrome.

The decrease in FEV indicates an obstruction to the flow of air only from the association of decrease of bronchial permeability index. This fact appear in the case of shrinking of the airway caliber or decreasing the amount of elastic fibers.

If the FEV is low and the Tiffeneau index is of normal, or even increased, the patient suffers from restrictive ventilatory dysfunction.

In a diffuse interstitial lung disease in which the lung volume is reduced but pulmonary elasticity is increased, FEV is not changed but the Tiffeneau index is upper limit of normal or increased.

Also, concomitant severe drop in FEV and Tiffeneau index often indicates pulmonary hyperinflation and arterial hypoxemia together with hypercapnia. The result is decreased exercise capacity.

Inspiratory volume per one second (FIV, or FIV_1) has the same functional meaning as FEV, except that is executed during inspiration.

The normal ratio between FEV and FIV is 0,8.

With IVF can be diagnose upper airway obstructive processes undetectable on clinical criteria.

Ventilation of rest per minute (VRM) is the total amount of air that enters the lungs in a minute at rest (equal to the volume of air exhaled in the same unit of time). VRM is the product of current volume and respiratory rate, has values of 6-8 liters/minute and can be calculated from spirogram. Elevated values are registered during exercise (exercise ventilation).

Maximum ventilation (MV) corresponds to the limit value that can increase ventilation per minute, VM being obtained only volunteer for a short period of time. It can be calculated in two ways:
- direct VM in spirometry with fast paper: the patient is asked to breathe for 15 seconds as it can deeply and quickly, and the amount of ventilation per 15 seconds be multiplied by 4
- indirect VM , through product FEV times 30

It is considered pathological the followung values of spirometry tests:
- percentage decreases by more than 8% and for FEV and VC
- percentage decreases by more than 6% for the Tiffeneau index.

The residual volume (RV), total lung capacity (CPT) and functional residual capacity (FCR) can be assessed using a gas analyzer coupled with a spirograph.

The residual volume is increased in obstructive ventilatory dysfunction, emphysema, and decreased in diffuse pulmonary fibrosis or pulmonary stasis of cardiac origin.

Paraclinical examinations:

pneumotachography	Pneumotachography is used to determine CV, representing the recording of curve flow-time; it may be determined instantaneous ventilatory flow and functional vital capacity (FVC).
Examination of costovertebral statics and dynamics The Maccagno method	The cirtometric index is normal between 6-8 cm. The method was developed by F. Maccagno and consists of graphic recording of the thoracic perimeter, easured at appendix xifoid level, in forced inhale and exhale, using a lead tape, 80 cm long and 1 cm wide.

was amended by Hreniuc who conceived chest symmetry index and index of parietal mobility	Chest symmetry index (CSI right/left) represents the ratio of sectional area between left and right hemithorax and is 1 in case of a perfectly symmetrical thorax (normal value is between 0.95 and 1.05). The supraunitary values indicated the left costal wall retraction and the subunitary ones the opposite situation.
	Parietal mobility index (PMI right/left) represents the ratio of the maximum inspiratory area and minimum expiratory area, normal values ranging from 15 for the basal level to 17 for pectoral level. Low values indicate retraction of costal wall.
Maximum capacity of effort (replaces exercise testing)	The Skibinski index is the ratio between voluntary inspiratory apnea x vital capacity and heart rate x100 and has values between 20 and 30, indicating efficiency of hematosis.

Silverman score is used to evaluate neonatal respiratory distress - tachypnea, cyanosis, respiratory signs of struggle.

If a score below 5 is recommended one physical therapy session per day, and for a score of more than 5 are recommended two sessions per day.

Although chest physiotherapy techniques in children requiring ventilator support (percussion, vibration) have been implemented in most clinics of neonatology in the world, their effectiveness remains debatable [5].

Cap. 7. Effort testing for the respiratory apparatus

Those tests explores respiratory apparatus ability to adapt to effort, being preceded by a clinical examination of the cardiovascular system and an electrocardiogram.

Effort testing		
objectives	contraindications	
	absolute	relative
- establishing the diagnosis - objectifying of patient accusations, especially dyspnoea - elucidation of the mechanism by which the ability to adapt to exercise is limited (fan, cardio-circulatory, muscular) - evaluation of the severity of functional disability - directing therapy and assessment of therapeutic effect - assessing disease progression - individualization of the recovery program - assessing physical performance development of a healthy subject subjected to great physical efforts - assessing the physical performance of subjects exposed to respiratory hazards - providing the operative risk factors (chest surgery)	- myocardial infarction with age less than 5 days - acute febrile illness - congestive heart failure - unstable angina - acute myocarditis - acute pericarditis - refractory hypertension (SBP> 250 mm Hg DBP> 120 mmHg) - close aortic stenosis - severe obstructive cardiomyopathy - dissecting aortic aneurysm - respiratory failure of pulmonary origin $PaO_2<40$	- myocardial infarction with age under 4 weeks - atrioventricular block degree II or III - aortic valvular disease - resting ECG abnormalities - resting tachycardia (heart rate above 120/min) - ventricular arrhythmias - atrial flutter - severe electrolyte disturbances - thromboembolism, including MET - orthopedic disorders - aneurysms - neurological disorders affecting adaptation to exercise - uncompensated diabetes - epilepsy - refractory asthma

		mmHg, $PaCO_2>70$ mmHg, FEV <30% of theoretical value	

Indications to interrupt effort testing		
general signs and symptoms	EKG signs	cardiovascular signs
- anginal type chest pain - severe dyspnoea - dizziness, asthenia - anxiety, confusion, incoordination, headache, delirium - suddenly appeared pallor and sweating - nausea, vomiting - cyanosis - muscular cramps	- signs of myocardial ischemia (ST descending or horizontal, subsided at least 1 mm, T-wave inversion, the occurrence of the Q wave) - polymorph supraventricular extrasystoles - paroxysmal ventricular tachycardia - atrial fibrillation occurring during exercise - atrioventricular block degree II or III - right or left bundle-branch block induced by exercise	- decrease of SBP below the resting value - decrease in TAS by more than 20 mm Hg after a normal growth to effort adaptation - SBP above 300 mmHg or DBP above 140 mmHg

A number of factors such as the nutritional, psychological, climatic, and of course physical condition of the subject influences effort testing.

Pathological factors influencing effort testing		
respirators	cardiovascular	musculoskeletal
- gas exchange disorder - mechanical ventilation disorder	- ischemic heart disease - valvulopathies	- neuromuscular disorders -musculoskeletal

- ventilation adjustment disorders - deficit of respiratory muscles	- myocarditis - pulmonary heart - pulmonary vascular disease - peripheral vascular disease	disorders

Stress testing of the respiratory function is accomplished by means of ergometers.

types of ergometers	features
treadmill	- enable the provision of muscular effort by an usual activity - walking - effort can be varied by changing the speed band or inclination from the horizontal (or both simultaneously) - the size of the effort (the mechanical work) can not be determined precisely because it depends on the patient's weight, type of gait and steplength - the effort is expressed in km/h and the slope of the band in percentage degrees
bicycle ergometer	- bicycle ergometer enables dosing of effort, because increasing resistance to pedaling and pedaling frequency can be changed - another advantage is that the mechanical work does not depend on the subject's weight - because of the relative immobility of the chest and arms cycloergometer, compared with treadmill, offers better conditions for the measurement of blood pressure and blood and breath collection - the effort performed is generally lower than on the treadmill (where come into action more muscle groups), and consequently the maximum intake of O_2 is about 7% lower - mechanical work done at cycloergometer is expressed in 1 kg/m - the power is expressed into mechanical work per unit of time (kg/meters/minute) or Watts (1W = 6.12 kg/m/minute); - the energy consumed is assessed on the basis of O_2 consumption

Are used the following types of exercise tests:

protocol	features
exercise tests at constant power (rectangular effort)	- the effort last 5-8 minutes at the same power - then, depending on the results, the test was repeated (after a pause of 30 min to 2 hours) - repetition is done at upper or lower power, while maintaining constant break - occupational medicine are used to estimate adaptation to a certain amount of effort - are also useful for evaluating the therapeutic progress (in terms of adaptation to effort)
exercise test to progressive growing power (tests in steps or triangular effort)	- duration of an exercise is between 8 - 15 minutes - power of effort is increased at predetermined intervals between 1 and 6 minutes - at the end of each interval takes place measurement of power - the test continues until it has reached maximum volume of oxygen or until pathological signs - this test is used more frequently in order to determine the strength at which the maximum volume of oxygen is reached (estimate the functional aerobic deficit for pathological cases) and maximum heart rate

Technical variants of the effort test	
Test of effort	mode for carrying out/followed parameters
Triangular effort on cycloergometer	- bicycle ergometer test is performed on a subject who breathes through the mouth (nose pension) by a piece fitted to a valve system with very low resistance to flow, so that the individual breathes atmospheric air and exhalation to be made to a bellows communicating via several openings to the outside - the expiratory part of the device (the bellows) is equipped with a flow sensor (from a pneumotachograph) fitted with an integrator of volume - the expired air (from the bellows) is

	sucked out continuously with a pump and then passed through the O_2 and CO_2 analyzer - recorded parameters: expired current volume (ECV), respiratory frequency/min, O_2 and CO_2 concentration in expired air - data processing shows the collection of O_2/min and the elimination of CO_2/min - after 5-6 minutes of breathing at rest, blood was collected from radial artery by catheter and determine PaO_2, $PaCO_2$, and pH - pe baza constantelor de mai sus se calculează parametrii echilibrului acido-bazic - other physiological constants are blood pressure and pulse rate, plus recording the ECG - as a manner of work, is started at cycloergometer, by pedaling without electrical resistance,and then introduced progressively increasing resistance - at intervals of 2 minutes power of effort becomes larger by 25 W down to use the maximum quantity of oxygen, in normal individuals duration of the test being 15 minutes - during the test are monitored physiological constants mentioned above, and in minutes 5, 10, 15, arterial blood is collected for determination of blood gas and acid-base balance evaluation
Triangular effort with increasing dosage of 100 kg /m/min	- 100 kg/m/min corresponds to an intake of O_2 about 200 ml/min higher - the test lasts until achievement maximum volume of O_2 - the test is limited by the following symptoms: intense dyspnea or cramps First period of the test - depending on exercise capacity, the test takes between 4 - 20 minutes The second period of the test consists of two rectangular efforts made at 1/3 and

	2/3 of maximum power achieved during triangular effort. - in the case of the above is evaluated the taking of O_2 and CO_2 elimination in steady state conditions, the alveolar ventilation, the ratio between the distribution and total volume The third period of the test includes O_2 and CO_2 measurements from arterial blood.
Cycloergometer constant effort to a minimum of 5 minutes	This test is used where the patient condition does not permit other samples effort. It is calculated current maximum ventilation power (or current FEV), PaO_2 at rest and after 5 minutes of effort. Cycloergometer constant effort to a minimum of 5 minutes is used for: - diagnosing latent pulmonary failure, in which case, PO_2 is normal at rest, but decreases by at least 5 mm Hg with the effort - identify the cause of a manifest lung failure; thus, a pulmonary insufficiency at rest by abnormal distribution of ventilation is characterized by hypoxemia at rest and increased PaO_2 during exercise, increased hypoxemia effort to produce a discrete hypercapnia (or worsening of preexisting one) are signs of depletion of functional reserves, and effort interruption because of dyspnea after 1-3 minutes means a drastic reduction of these reserves
The walking test	In this test is assessed the distance traveled by the patient in 12 minutes of normal march without stopping. The test follows the occurrence and severity of dyspnea, for patients with very small functional reserve.

The maximum volume of oxygen, or the removal (intake) of O_2 (expressed in ml/min or mmol/min) from the blood conducting pulmonary perfusion is equal to the oxygen consumption at the cellular level.

Prelevation of oxygen increases with power of effort up to a maximum representing maximal oxygen intake (beyond which, however would increase the power of effort, O_2 intake remains constant). Maximum oxygen intake defines capacity to adapt to effort and power of effort on wich it has been achieved represents maximal aerobic power. To a higher value than maximal aerobic power the effort can not continue than a few minutes, and at a lower value of power the effort may be extended inversely proportional to respective value (% of maximum aerobic power).

Since interindividual variations are very high exercise capacity can be estimated more accurately by the maximum supported power (MSP), defined as the maximal aerobic power on wich respiratory gas exchange still occurs in steady state. MSP has values of approximately 100 W at untrained individuals and at least 200 watts at trained ones. Typically, in patients, it is estimated maximum volume of oxygen that is limited by symptoms: intense dyspnoea, muscle cramps, joint pain, fatigue.

To ensure the respiratory test to effort deployment, cardiovascular monitoring is required during exercise (heart rate and, intermittently, blood pressure, and perform electrocardiogram to capture any rhythm disturbances and irregularities of ST segment).

Patients with chronic lung disease presents some peculiarities of adaptation to exercise, summarized below.

physiological constants/modified tests/pathological changes	conditions/clinical significance/tests/pathophysiological mechanism
decrease O_2 intake and also the maximum value of the maximum power supported	means a lower ability to adapt to exercise
increase in respiratory gas exchange ratio above 1 and of serum lactate more than 4 mmol/l in a small or medium-power effort	means an insufficient intake of O_2 to the active muscles; the causes can be deficits in ventilation or respiratory failure by abnormal transport or use of cellular O_2
maximum ventilation/minute lower than the predicted one	the disorder characterizes situations in which exercise capacity is limited by poor ventilation. In the case of severe obstructive ventilatory dysfunction, with greatly increase of respiratory labor, increased ventilation/minute does not provide an additional intake of oxygen than in breathing muscles

respiratory type during exercise changed in patients with obstructive ventilatory dysfunction	- the disorder is characterized by increased flow resistance especially during expiratory phase - increased breathing results in shortness of breath and increased labor of fans muscles; consequently appears dyspnoea - in patients with restrictive ventilatory dysfunction the increase in ventilation is based on breathing frequency, thus facilitate the work of the respiratory muscles; in the case of this pathophysiological mechanism dyspnea occurs due to hypoxemia
decrease at effort of O_2 ventilation equivalent	meaning is improving the distribution of ventilation-perfusion ratios with increasing minute ventilation and cardiac output
lowering at the effort of partial pressure of arterial O_2, possibly associated with increased partial pressure of CO_2	- has the pathophysiological significance of a failure to adapt ventilation and circulation for additional metabolic needs induced by exercise - decrease in arterial O_2 partial pressure below 55 mmHg requires effort off - obstructive ventilatory dysfunction in patients with severe alveolar ventilation can not ensure the elimination of CO2 during exercise, and as a result occurs hypercapnia and respiratory acidosis
decrease in alveolar-arterial gradient of O_2 during effort	it has a positive predictive value, excluding a disorder of alveolar-capillary diffusion membrane
increase in ratio between the current volume and respiratory dead space during exercise	- the disorder appears in case of obstructive ventilatory dysfunction or at patients with pulmonary vasculitis - the meaning is a ventilation proportionally higher than the perfusion - is often associated a pulmonary arterial hypertension
decrease of the blood pressure of O_2 of at least 5 mm Hg at the effort, with simultaneous reduction of	the modification occurs in disorders of alveolar-capillary transfer through the membrane and is the result of diffuse interstitial pneumopathies or atrophic

the CO_2 pressure if the effort continues	primitive emphysema

Causes of limiting exercise capacity identified by testing of respiratory function at effort	
etiology	functional signs
of cardiovascular origin	lowering the maximum volume of oxygen, normal ventilatory reserve, decreased intake of O_2 to the end of the effort, increased heart rate
of ventilatory origin	a symptom-limited decrease in maximal oxygen volume and a reduced ventilatory reserve

Cap. 8. Physical therapy for patients with respiratory diseases

Respiratory physical therapy includes the following methods/steps/objectives: relaxation, postural drainage, corrective gymnastics, respiratory gymnastics itself or respiratory rehabilitation, training for dosed effort, education of cough, education of speaking, occupational therapy.

Relaxation

indications for relaxation	curative mechanisms
crisis prevention and stopping at paroxysmal asthma sufferers	reducing emotional triggers wich triggers hyperactivity with bronchospasm, dyspnea and cough in patients with asthma
	removes a number of inhibitors conditions which disrupt ventilatory control
decrease the need for sympathomimetic in asthmatics	rebalancing respiratory muscle tone
improving psycho-emotional state, decrease of anxiety	decline in demand for O_2 and CO_2 production

Relaxation technique called "reciprocal inhibition" is particularly effective for combating anxiety.

Relaxation techniques		
	features	subcategories
"extrinsic" relaxation	relaxation is mediated by an external factor, which creates a dependency condition of the patient, another drawback is its passive position relative to the therapy	pharmacotherapy (sedatives, neuroplegics, muscle-relaxants drugs)
		sedative and muscle relaxant massage
		different massage and vibratory massage apparatus
		hypnosis
"intrinsic" relaxation	- the method is autonomous, even in the event of initial intervention	Hatha-Yoga
		Zen
		Soufis
		Jacobson method

	of the therapist - is the only method that realize reciprocal inhibition mental sphere - muscle	Psychological current like to implement "type central" relaxation techniques. They are based on imaginative mental self control. The objective is to achieve peripheral relaxation, thus being influenced visceral paratonia.
		Maccagno method
		Muscular relaxation techniques. These include rhythmic gymnastics, artistic gymnastics, collective gymnastics with totally free, not imposed movements, done in various positions, with breath awareness. This includes the Parow method, according to which the patient sits in bed 20 minutes, breathing as easily as possible (unforced), and exhaling with saying a "hush" or "pfff", thereby achieving overall muscle relaxation.

Postural drainage

Posture is a very important process for the management of patients with respiratory diseases, in fact they instinctively adopting certain posts that facilitate ventilation.

Category of posture	Features/method
Relaxing and breathing facilitating postures	The facilitating upright posture for the big dyspneic found in crisis is back against the wall, slightly kyphosis spine, torso bent forward and shoulders slightly "fallen" (arms hanging). The legs are slightly bent at the knee, the position inducing relaxation of the abdominal muscles. It can also be used a facilitating position, from orthostatism: the patient has the trunk slightly flexed and head supported on the

	forearms (variant - trunk flexed and resting on a higher level, with support on forearms). There are relaxing supine positions, ie supine with the flap of the bed elevated at 45 degrees. The head, not the shoulders, rests on a small pillow. The arms are in abduction at 30 - 40 degrees and the forearms are resting on two pillows on both sides of the body. Under the thighs and knees is placed another pillow that bend easily the hips and knees. The legs are supported on a support. Relaxing in seated positions is characterized by the fact that the trunk is leaning forward (which facilitates diaphragmatic breathing movements by reducing intra-abdominal pressure), with forearms resting on the knees. They indicated especially in patients undergoing thoracic surgery and have the effect of relieving dyspnea. As alternatives exist 'mohammedan" position and seated on the bed or floor with knees bent over the plants on the ground, arms hanging at his sides, slightly bent trunk. There is also the posture: sitting on shins and heels with hands on the thighs and the trunk slightly bent.
bronchial drainage postures	For the recovery of patients with chronic pulmonary diseases the main objective is evacuation of secretions, which is carried out by means of gravity, based on the gradient level. Drainage positions correspond to obstructed bronchial segments; must be ensuring the sloping drain from the respective area to the trachea. Postural drainage facilitators factors are stimulating expiratory flow (slowdown inspiring to avoid aspiration of secretions) and external chest vibrations. Expiratory flow can be increased by exerting external

	pressure on the chest. Regarding external chest vibrations, have the highest efficiency the frequency of 100-500 Hz. If the patient can not cough and bronchial aspiration can not be performed, is waived to bronchial drainage positions.

Program for home care of patients with bronchial obstruction

Morning and evening is executed the following exercise program [6]:

Exercise I	It runs from sitting position. It comprises five stations, each maintained 10-15 seconds: 1. Standing straight up 2. Right lateral trunk bending, at 45^0 3. Left lateral trunk bending at 45^0 4. Posterior trunk bending, at 30^0 5. Trunk bends above at 45^0
Exercise II	Made of decubitus includes two posts, lasting 10-15 seconds each: 1. supine position (without pillow) 2. ventral decubitus
Exercise III	Execution is made from lateral decubitus, 4 positions, lasting 10-15 seconds each. 1. The patient positioned in the left lateral decubitus position with a small pillow under the head. 2. The patient perform a pivot on the left shoulder, with turning as much as possible in front of the right shoulder and torso. 3 and 4. The patient reverses movements (in the right lateral decubitus).
Exercise IV	The patient is positioned in the ventral decubitus with a pillow under the lower abdomen and head resting on forearms crossed before; the posture is maintained 10-15 s.
Exercise V	Maintain 20 seconds the following posture: in the bed tilted at 15 degrees (Trendelenburg), supine with a small pillow under the buttocks and knee flexed to 90 degrees.
Exercise VI	It consists of 2 positions, 11-15 s each, made from

	Trendelenburg. 1. The left lateral decubitus position with a pillow under the hips and chest basis. 2. The right lateral decubitus.
Exercise VII	It includes 4 positions, lasting 10-15 seconds each, bed being positioned as in the previous exercise. 1. dorsal decubitus. 2. rotation of the torso to the left with pivoting the left shoulder, right shoulder in this way reaching 45 degrees. The legs remain stretched with the fingers up. 3. resume supine. 4. the same practice as in point 2, except that the rotation is clockwise.
Exercise VIII	The exercise is executed to the end of the program and aims the drainage of large bronchi. The patient is positioned in ventral decubitus, crosswise the bed, with basin and legs on the bed and trunk bent toward the floor (makes an angle of about 45 degrees) and head resting on his hands placed on the floor. Posture is maintained at least 3 minutes, until 20 minutes. The patient will have a glass for secretions.
Variants of exercises to drain the large bronchi	- the time devoted to such exercises is variable depending on the patient from tens of seconds to several minutes - are associated vibrations and percussions of the chest - first variant: from prone position, the patient is connected to a strap of the middle on a special table and the chest, wich sits on a fly tables portion, is drooping so that the trunk makes an angle of 60-70 degrees with the basin and lower limbs - version II: the same as above, but lying on the side, in which case the inclination of the trunk will be only 45 degrees - variant III: a variant of "goat", the patient is standing next to a pedestal which reaches the basin, on this bend the trunk how much can, abdomen supported by the goat and shoulders on some stops
As a general indication, after each posture, patient breathe deeply several times, after which coughed several times in purpose to	

> expectoration.
> At the end of each positioning, for 1 minute, will be executed tapping on (for viscous sputum) or vibration (for fluids sputum) above the drained segment.

The following adjunctive and complementary procedures are recommended for special clinical cases:
- using modified drainage postures
- bronchodilators 10-15 minutes prior to the implementation of the exercise program in patients with obstructive phenomena

Other indications:
- bronchial drainage is done before the meal
- the process is conducted once or several times a day, as required
- whole lung drainage should not last more than 30-45 minutes, during which alternates the important postures, each lasting 5-10 minutes.
- areas with the most pronounced dullness are drained first
- after draining are given aerosol antibiotics and corticosteroids

Indications to perform postural drainage	Indications to perform postural drainage in modified positions	Contraindications for maneuvers to chest percussion and vibration	Therapeutic effects of postural drainage
- medical or surgical emergencies such as respiratory hemoptysis, pneumothorax, intrabronhic foreign body, pulmonary embolism, pulmonary edema - uncooperative patient	- dyspnoea - associated cardiac pathology - hiatal hernia - age of the patient - obesity - postoperative period	- chest pain - chest trauma - pneumothorax - pleurisy - empyema - upper abdominal pathology	- increasing the forced vital capacity and peak expiratory flow in patients with cystic fibrosis and chronic bronchitis - FEV increase in young patients

Corrective gymnastics

Gymnastics has a special role in correcting respiratory pathology. Thus, patients with chronic obstructive pulmonary disease presents the following musculoskeletal disorders, which are part of the causes of respiratory disease or its consequences: muscle contractures (98% of cases), stiffness of thoracic joints (92% of cases), dorsal kyphosis (89% of cases), dorsal scoliosis (61% of cases), paravertebral and rib pain (76% of cases), muscle hypotony (52% of cases) high shoulder (76% of cases).

These can be improved through specific exercises. Gymnastics correction may have prophylactic character, in which case take the form of collective therapy. Preparing for kinesiotherapy is through physiotherapy.

Methodologies of corrective gymnastics at the gym [6]		
Gymnastics at the gym	Aquatic gymnastics	Manipulations (Maigne)
It can be performed at medical physical culture halls, or in the patient's home. Goals are correcting pathological curvature of the neck and head, shoulder, scapula, dorsal and lumbar spine position. Emphasis will be placed on abdominal breathing, diaphragm and transverse abdominal reeducation. **Exercises for the reeducation of diaphragm** 1. The exercise, which require especially the back of the diaphragm, runs	Aquatic gymnastics can be done individually or in groups. Compared to the gym, the aquatic gymnastics has the following advantages: - water temperature (standardized between 32-36 degrees) has analgesic and relaxing effect - the heat has an action of increasing the muscle suppleness - movements can be facilitated by the hydrostatic pressure of water, or it can be used as	Restrictive functional dysfunction benefit from the therapeutic effects of manipulation. Blockages in the costovertebral or posterior intervertebral joints manifested by local pain, spontaneous and at pressure, pain irradiated metameric or on posterior branch of rachidian nerve, stiff of thoracic and sometimes lumbar segment of spine, low mobility of the chest and pain at insertion of large and small oblique muscles or of the diaphragm, or occurring in patients with chronic pulmonary diseases benefit from these therapeutic procedures. Other therapeutic procedures wich are

from supine with the knee flexed and a load of 5 kg placed on the abdomen; patient inspires lifting the abdominal wall and expires with his depression. Alternatively, to enhance exhale, lift the knees to the chest during this phase of respiration. 2. The exercise runs from prone position with the abdomen resting on a pillow. On the basis of the chest is placed a minimum 2 and maximum weight of 9 kg. From this position the patient performs abdominal breaths, thus being requested especially the front of the diaphragm. 3. From sitting position, torso tilted slightly forward and your knees slightly apart, the patient performs abdominal breaths. 4. For a hemidiaphragm, from lateral decubitus position with a pillow under	opposite resistance	useful in case of costovertebral blockages are heat, massage, electrotherapy, ultrasound, diadynamic currents, ultrashort waves, local infiltration with corticosteroids and lidocaine 1%, medical gymnastics.

the base of hemithorax and homolateral leg semiflected, the patient is made to execute abdominal breaths.

5. For toning the diaphragm and oblique muscles, from lateral decubitus position, legs slightly bent, the patient execute a speed exhale, pronouncing the letter "f". As an alternative, the patient can perform a deep inspiration followed by two quick exhalations. The exercise is repeated 5 times.

6. Breathing exercises (inspir with resistance) for toning the diaphragm: abdomen relaxed, inhale is made saying a sucked "f", or "s" with the tongue on upper incisors with a finger between parted lips. As an alternative, the patient inspires one nostril, pressing a finger on the other side.

7. Simultaneously with the diaphragm toning is made abdominal muscle re-education. Thus, supine with the knee flexed, the patient raises the trunk, upper limbs outstretched and passed above the knees. As a more difficult alternative, chest lifting is performed with hands behind your head. Also for rectus abdominis, in supine, lift the legs with knees straight. 8. Also for abdominal muscles - big and small oblique, in supine position, with one knee bent, lift and turn in homolateral direction the trunk, upper limbs stretched sideways. To increase the difficulty, the exercise can be performed with hands behind the head. 9. For the transverse muscle, from knee-elbow position, in exhale, strongly retracted abdomen.		

Maintain seconds.	3-5		

A variant is breathing with hands placed on the abdomen to control pressure variations caused by movements of the diaphragm [7].

Cap. 9. Respiratory gymnastics

Reeducation of breath through gymnastics comprises a set of specific kinetic and analytical techniques aimed at stopping and then reversing the deterioration of respiratory function.

Goals are augmenting respiratory flows and volumes, reduction of ventilator mechanical labor (decreased resistance to dynamic flow and/or increased chest compliance), increase respiratory muscle tone, optimization of respiratory rhythm.

Exercises for directing the air to the upper respiratory tract

The normal development and rehabilitation of respiratory muscles have like first condition acquiring or restoring right inspiration on the nose, in that way developing breathing muscles and skeleton of rib cage at growing child.

Inspiratory muscle toning exercises	- alternative breathing : the patient inspires trough one nostril, compressing the other with the finger - interrupted inspires, imitating trailing - inspires with rhythmic beating the wings of the nose with the fingers
Exercises to facilitate nasal inspiration in the case of dyspnea	- slight towed with thumb and index in the nasal groove during inspiration - active dilation of nostrils in inspiration
Indications for expiration	Patients with obstructive syndrome will perform oral exhalation in order to reduce flow resistance; the exception is the low ambient temperature. Alternatively, there are "tight-lipped breathing," in wich case the patient out through the mouth with tight lips or pronouncing *h, s, f, s, pf,* thus being prevented bronchial collapse.
Music therapy	It is a method that has as principle a correct posture and training during the singing of deep inspirations followed by short apnea.

Reeducation of costal breathing

For coastal respiratory rehabilitation is applied an opposite resistance to movement of coasts.

Techniques [6]	purposes
The hands of physiotherapist are positioned on the desired area with fingers along the coast, and the patient is asked to perform a full exhale. During this time, hands creates a pressure that increases progressively as the end approaches of expiration, thereby breathing muscles being put under tension. Inspir that follow will be under resistance, leading to increased muscle tension. At the end of the inspir manual pressure will gradually weaken so that the chest is released.	awareness of coastal movement, after that the patient being able to execute the technique in the respiratory rehabilitation program
alternatively, the resistance is created by means of sandbags from 8 to 12 kg.	increase the amplitude of inspir and facilitate expiration, thus being increased ventilation underlying lung area
use of straps to create resistance	regional inspiratory muscle strength development

Technical details of the costal breathing rehabilitation in different regions [6]	
Reeducation of pulmonary apex regions	1. With the physical therapist standing at the patient's head with his thumb on the breastbone and fingers to the armpit, and the patient supine with the neck and head in rectitude, will be atrenate both regions of pulmonary apex or only one through active resistance. After a while the patient can work from sitting position. 2. In case of evolutional injury of apex region of the left lung, with the patient in supine, head bent to the left, the right hand under the neck, left arm along the body, the physiotherapist will apply manual pressure in the region of right lung

	apex. Concomitantly the left hand of physiotherapist tried to completely block the expansion of the lungs during inspiration in the apex region of the left lung.
Reeducation of axillary lung sector	The patient is positioned in the lateral decubitus position, with his head bent toward the bed and above arm in abduction. Physiotherapist places his hands in the armpit and performs pressure during exhalation, reducing it to its end. Alternatively, the patient may be placed in the seating position.
Reeducation of low and medium coastal regions	Position of the patient is supine with the head flexed and supported by a pillow, upper limbs along the body, and physiotherapist hands exercise compression of the chest base, with the thumb on the center line (lower coastal training will be associated with diaphragmatic breathing).
Reeducation of lower thoracic breathing	For this purpose is used a strap of huckaback, wide 8-10 cm and 1.50 m long, fitted at the ends with two handles crossed at the base of the chest so that each hand of physiotherapist can control the pressure of homolateral hemithorax. In the expiration, if the patient moves away his hands, the thoracic base is circularly compressed by the strap (in inspiration the traction gradually weakens). If it is desired a unilaterally lower cost zone entrainment, the patient is placed in lateral decubitus, with the head in low position and positioned above the upper limb in order to open the hemithorax (aspect that can be enhanced by placing a pillow under the hemithorax base). The physical therapist will perform manual pressure on hemithorax above. Another option is the unilateral training of the thoracic base through strap positioned as for both bases. The patient performs a lateral deviation in the opposite direction as for hemithorax which is intended to be treated. Carry out an exhale against the backdrop of traction of both ends of the strap, then an inspir during which, using the strap, is made a hemithorax compression, weakening towards the

	end of this phase of breathing.
Reeducation of posterior rib	With the patient placed in prone position, the therapist places his hands on coastal posteroinferiorly areas exerting the required strength for respiratory reeducation .
Reeducation of affected hemithorax by the patient	The execution takes place in lateral decubitus with a pillow placed under the lumbar region and head lower than chest to cause "openness" of the hemithorax. In a first time, in inspir, outstretched arm rotates with the trunk backwards, eyes and head following the movement of the hand, and during the second time, executed in expiration, arm returns to the torso, continuing the race beyond the edge of the bed, while trunk rotation toward its plan. Reeducation from sitting position can be done from two basic positions. The first involves supporting hands on hips and rotate the arm back during inspiration. Simultaneously occurs twisting of torso in the same direction; the look and head follows the hand movement. During exhalation, the movement is reversed. In the second base position, a hand is placed on top of the head and the other resting on the thigh. Inspir is accompanied by rotation of the trunk, arm and head towards hemithorax wich wants to be treated. In the expiration the patient returns to the basic position and the reverse rotation is performed with bending of the trunk.

Diaphragmatic breathing reeducation

To increase the amplitude of motion of the diaphragm and thus alleviate fatigue to abdominal breathing, is used resistance training against the diaphragm (sandbags), beginning with 2 kg , following the progressive loading of up to 10 kg, which is placed on the abdomen.

It should be made a difference between patients with lung restrictive disease and those with obstructive syndrome because if at first it may increase resistance even up to double the standard above, in the second category loading must be relatively small, otherwise the rectus abdominis muscle contraction in the lower position blocks the diaphragm (antigravitational reflex).

Training of the diaphragm	given that in the forced expiration increase tension in the back diaphragm, to its muscle toning is recommended Trendelenburg posture.
	jerky inspire on the nose
	inspire by one nostril or mouth through a tube made of variable length and diameter
	Method Pescher uses two jars, A and B, connected to each other by a tube, jar A containing water. The patient can train inspiratory muscles, inspiring from the jar B until water movement in A, or expiratory muscles, exhaling in the jar A until it is emptied of water. In this way are toned not only pillar of the diaphragm but also abdominal muscles.
Diaphragm-abdominal training associated with exhalation exercises	To recover the elasticity of diaphragm can be associated diaphragm-abdominal training (with a frequency of 5-10 minutes, 3 times a day) with an exercise intended to reduce resistances in expiration (breathing with tight lips).
Training of an hemidiaphragm	One proceeds in homo lateral position with the head on a pillow and arm sitting on the chest. In this mode is blocked heterolateral chest expansion. The physical therapist approaches the patient's homo costoiliac space manually during exhalation, pressing in and up, and in breathing out leaving the hemidiaphragm free. Thus intra-abdominal pressure will bomb the half of diaphragm.
	The exercise above can run during apnea after inspiration, in which case therapy is indicated for bag bottom pleural adhesions, because of the low position of the hemidiaphragm during inspiration.

Monitoring and coordination of breathing

To correct respiratory deficiency is needed a new system of breathing (ventilation must be guided in terms of the magnitude relative to effort), which will depend on functional testing and condition of the patient.

The main objective of respiratory reeducation consists of a slow respiratory rate, which will be carried out in stages, without forcing the patient (therapeutic session is stopped at the occurrence of discomfort).

This decrease in the frequency of respiratory movements is down to 10-12 breaths/minute, 4-6 breaths for one step. Ideal is the correlation with heart rate, breathe in and out occurring every 3-6 pulses (breathing exercises are under the control of peripheral pulse).

This gives decreased respiratory rate and current volume increase, particularly needed in obstructive respiratory disorders. For the restricted type diseases, compliance while decreases concomitant with increasing intrapulmonarily volume; should therefore be carried pulmonary ventilation at lower current volumes.

Relationship between respirators times and length of the breaks between them are important in the respiratory rehabilitation because respiration rate reduction can be achieved by prolonging time of breathing, by prolonging pauses between them, or both possibilities.

Reeducation of obstructive breathing dysfunctions requires decline in the inhale/exhale from 1/1.2 as is normally to 1/2 - 1/2.5 (the patient exhales double enduring). It can rithmah breathing pulse, from time equals respirators. Thus, on 2 - 3 - 4 heartbeat, increases expiratory time to double the number of heart beats.

In patients with sequels after pleurisy, is recommended a pause after inspiration. Its role is to achieve a "posture" to combat air pleural adhesions. After inspiration apnea requires gradual increase of exhalation to a maximum - 2 times. And after exhale the patient can take a break, as a stimulus of the cough reflex.

Controlling the flow of air includes both respiratory rate, the volumes of air mobilized, the ratio between respiratory times and the speed of the inspiratory air stream in and out. Given that chronic obstructive pulmonary disease patient has an increased frequency of respiratory movements and prints high speed airflow (which increases respiratory mechanical labor and consequently worsens poor oxygenation of tissues), rehabilitation of breath will follow acquiring an inspir and an expire slow, extended. Among reeducation methods of expire is "blowing the candle" - the patient, first sitting then in orthostatism, blowing out a candle placed on a support located at the mouth level, at a distance of 15 - 25 cm. The aim is only to bend flame, not extinguished it, all during expiration. With training progression moves away the candle growing. Another option for directing controlled the breathing out is to expire through a rubber tube, glass or plastic in a 1 liter glass with some amount of water, watching as the liquid surface bubbles appear and break rhythmically equal and continuous; training progression is determined by the increase of the water level in the bottle [6]. This method has the advantage of avoiding the installation of dynamic bronchial compression.

Respiratory air flow control can be implemented gradually by following mental inspiration and expiration. The desire is that they are executed quietly.

Control of breathing during exercise is particularly important in patients with cardiorespiratory diseases, especially conditions with very low functional respiratory capacity or carrying out an intense and sustained effort (low duration). In a first stage, the patient must inspire before movement and expire the whole duration. Subsequently breathing will be monitored during walking, as follows: inspire one step and expires on 2 steps, then gradually increase the number of steps in wich is done the expiration. The inspire is done when climbing a step and the expire on two steps. The duration of respiratory gymnastics sessions assisted by physiotherapist varies from 2 to 30 minutes, depending on exercise tolerance of the patient, the total duration of therapy being 3-6 months. The patient will perform respiratory gymnastic exercises whole life, morning and evening, even during the lull of the disease.

Cap. 10. Tolerance of the respiratory patient to effort

Quality of life of respiratory patient is impaired by dyspnea. As a result, the effort required dosage. Dosage effort must take into account the fact that the appearance of hypoxemia is favored by the lactic acid. The evolution of respiratory flow during physical activity follows the cardiac output; over a certain amount of exercise intensity the ventilation no longer increase. In respiratory patients hypercapnia and metabolic acidosis occur at much lower values of exercise intensity than in healthy individuals. Generally, patients with obstructive ventilatory dysfunction respond more difficult to exercise (this type of response is directly proportional to the rate of CO_2 removal from the lungs) than those with restrictive or mixed dysfunction. In these patients tachypnea occur even at low intensity efforts, and hypoxia due to respiratory muscle fatigue limit increase of respiratory flow. The exercise is felt as discomfort, the physical activity being restricted. In patients with chronic obstructive pulmonary disease occurs an increase in end-expiratory level, accompanied by tachypnea, instead current volume is low (opposite situation compared to healthy individuals). Therefore, in order not to worsen ventilatory dysfunction, respiratory rehabilitation is due at low ventilatory rhythms. These considerations no longer apply if patients with COPD already have a low ventilator rhythm during exercise.

Regarding hypoxemia, this may occur during exercise in emphysematous COPD sufferers. In some chronic bronchitis (COPD type B) partial pressure of oxygen does not change during exercise, even may increase. Other patients with the same diagnosis shows a decrease of the respective parameter. Therefore it is tested first PO_2 in a standard effort, recovery program being established by the category in which it is the patient.

If at the test effort occurs hypoxaemia, will start with an intensity of effort less than that at which the test was positive. At the doctor indication may be administered oxygen.

Due to increased cardiac output and the degree of dissociation of oxyhemoglobin, the tissues of respiratory patient are better oxygenated during the effort.

Research in healthy subjects have shown that 6 weeks of electromiostimulation at low frequency (10 Hz) leads, in addition to increasing muscle volume and degree of pinnate, also to lowering blood pressure and increasing aerobic capacity, as an alternative to endurance training [8].

Similarly, functional aerobic deficit improves in respiratory patients who undergo a rehabilitation program based on exercise training.

As the intensity of effort become higher (supported without causing hypoxia) so it is considered that exercise tolerance has increased.

Clinical indicator of improving exercise tolerance is decreasing dyspnea of effort by at least 1 degree.

One problem is the possibility of triggering acute asthma during exercise. Expiratory volume in one second decreases less in asthmatics if the effort is put into a moist air (saturated).

Methodology of training to effort will be based on test results so on patient's exercise capacity and also blood gases ratio. The density and the intensity of effort will be determined by subsequent sequential testing that will highlight improving exercise capacity.

During the training shall be track the appearance (or enhancing) of dyspnea, tachypnea, cardiac arrhythmias, chest pain. The exercise will be discontinued if these signs and symptoms appear, or if the patient accuses discomfort.

Ergometer bicycle training	It has the advantage of opportunity of oxygen therapy, plus the dosage of a great power (mechanical labor/s); pedaling can be executed in the most convenient pace while maintaining constant power of effort. As a result, the dosage of exercise at the bicycle ergometer can be done either by increasing the intensity or the duration thereof.
Training on treadmill	The main advantage is that walking is a physiological action, consists of stereotypic movements, therefore there is the possibility of effective dosing the effort (due to automatism, walking on the treadmill requires a lower consumption of O_2 at the same intensity of effort to pedaling the bicycle ergometer, effort at the scale or squats). The variables according to is made the dosing of effort are scroll speed and slope. Training is initiated by walking on flat at increasing speeds and the maximum duration of 10 minutes. Follow walking on a slope of 10 degrees. Subsequently combine the two types of training with a break. The frequency is 2 times a week, with walking and scale exercises, performed at home.
Training at the scale	It uses the Master stairs stress test (scale of 2 steps, height 23 cm each).

Power of effort is calculated as follows:

Power (W) = 4/3 x patient weight (kg) x9,81x0,23x number of climbs per minute

Mechanical labor expressed in kg x meters/minute is calculated as follows:

Mechanical work (kg x m/min) = Weight (kg) x0,23x no. steps per minute/100

Usually sufferers of COPD with medium dysfunction can perform minimum 100 kg x m/min.
It starts at 1 minute/session, as the progression of training not exceeding the 10 minutes to avoid excessive consumption of oxygen.

Training by walking	Training by walking is useful to patients that and start mobilizing after an episode of acute respiratory failure (allows the port of oxygen mask). It can also be used for maintenance of the exercise capacity. For respiratory patients, therapeutic walking running only on flat ground. If the patient reaches 15 minutes without causing breathlessness or other pathological signs/symptoms are inserted short distance walking alerts rhythms (double or triple rhythm), intervals whose duration will gradually increase. The program will be individualized depending on the patient and condition. This type of training can be performed at home, ideally in an unpolluted environment.
Training at the pool	Training at the pool has the advantages of increasing hematosis (by homogenization of distribution in pulmonary circulation), limiting heat loss from the lining of the respiratory tract and thus stop the occurrence of bronchospasm, stimulate bronchial secretions evacuation, facilitate exhale through hydrostatic pressure, muscle toning.
Exercise training in other ways	This includes therapeutic sport and physical labor, both to be metered effort.

Recent research [9] showed that preoperative application of a specific protocol based on rehabilitation exercises of diaphragm for smokers, resulted in immediate improvement of respiratory muscle performance, which creates prerequisites for improving recovery after surgery in these patients.

Ventilatory disorders in children and adolescents may not only be due to chronic pulmonary disease, but also by neuromuscular diseases that comprise respiratory muscles too. Training of respiratory muscles at home with a duration of more than 6 months lead to improved respiratory muscle strength and peak cough flow [10].

The rehabilitation of patients with COPD requires respiratory muscles training, which is done through resistive training, pressure threshold loading and normocapnic hyperpnea, the most effective being inspiratory muscle training [11].

References

1. Pesut D, Ciobanu L, Nagorni-Obradovic L. Pneumologia. Pulmonary rehabilitation in chronic respiratory diseases-from goals to outcomes. 2008; 57(2):65-9.
2. Postolache PA, Petrescu OP. Respiratory Rehabilitation Effects On Bode Index Components And Correlation With Health-Related Quality Of Life In Copd, Chest, 2007;132(4_MeetingAbstracts):534b-534.
3. Holland AE, Wadell K, Spruit MA.Eur Respir Rev. How to adapt the pulmonary rehabilitation programme to patients with chronic respiratory disease other than COPD. 2013; 22(130):577-86.
4. Postolache Paraschiva. Farmacoterapie, vol I, Edit-Dan, 2004.
5. Hough JL, Flenady V, Johnston L, Woodgate PG. Chest physiotherapy for reducing respiratory morbidity in infants requiring ventilatory support.Cochrane Database Syst Rev 2008(3):CD006445.
6. Ocheana G. Kinetoterapia în afecțiuni respiratorii, Editura Pim, Iași, 2008.
7. Cigna, J.L. and Turner-Cigna, L.M. 2005. Rehabilitation for the home care patient with COPD, Home Healthcare Nurse, 23, 9, 578-584.
8. Deley G, Babault N. Could Low-Frequency Electromyostimulation Training be an Effective Alternative to Endurance Training? An Overview in One Adult. Journal of Sports Science & Medicine, 2014;13(2):444-450.
9. Galvan Carrie Chueiri Ramos, Cataneo Antônio José Maria. Effect of respiratory muscle training on pulmonary function in preoperative preparation of tobacco smokers. Acta Cir. Bras. 2007, 22(2): 98-104.
10. Rodríguez Iván, Zenteno Daniel, Manterola Carlos. Effects of home-based respiratory muscle training in children and adolescents with chronic lung disease. J. bras. pneumol. [Internet]. 2014 Dec [cited 2015 Nov 21] ; 40(6): 626-633. Available from: http://www.scielo.br/scielo.php?script=sci_arttext&pid=S1806-37132014000600626&lng=en. http://dx.doi.org/10.1590/S1806-37132014000600006.
11. Crisafulli E, Costi S, Fabbri LM, Clini EM. Respiratory muscles training in COPD patients. International Journal of Chronic Obstructive Pulmonary Disease. 2007;2(1):19-25.

Bibliography of the theme

1. Cambach W, Wagenaar RC, Koelman TW, van Keimpema AR, Kemper HC. The long-term effects of pulmonary rehabilitation in patients with asthma and chronic obstructive pulmonary disease: a research synthesis.

Arch Phys Med Rehabil. 1999 Jan; 80(1):103-11.
2. Jennifer A. Pryor and Ammani Prasad. Physiotherapy for Respiratory and Cardiac Problems, 4th Edition. Adults and Paediatrics. Churchill Livingstone, 2008.
3. Nellessen A, Hernandes NA, Pitta F. Physiotherapy and rehabilitative interventions in patients with chronic respiratory diseases: exercise and non-exercise treatment. Panminerva Med. 2013 Jun;55(2):197-209.

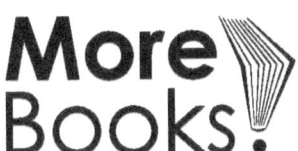
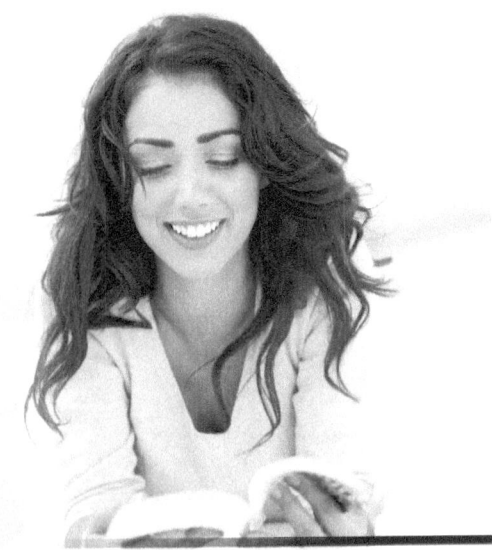

I want morebooks!

Buy your books fast and straightforward online - at one of the world's fastest growing online book stores! Environmentally sound due to Print-on-Demand technologies.

Buy your books online at
www.get-morebooks.com

Kaufen Sie Ihre Bücher schnell und unkompliziert online – auf einer der am schnellsten wachsenden Buchhandelsplattformen weltweit!
Dank Print-On-Demand umwelt- und ressourcenschonend produziert.

Bücher schneller online kaufen
www.morebooks.de

OmniScriptum Marketing DEU GmbH
Heinrich-Böcking-Str. 6-8
D - 66121 Saarbrücken
Telefax: +49 681 93 81 567-9

info@omniscriptum.com
www.omniscriptum.com

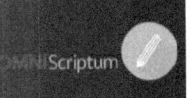

www.ingramcontent.com/pod-product-compliance
Lightning Source LLC
Chambersburg PA
CBHW031544210526
45464CB00003B/1137